Table of Contents

Endocrine Disorders

The endocrine system is a network of glands that produce and release hormones that help control many important body functions, including the body's ability to change calories into energy that powers cells and organs. The endocrine system influences how your heart beats, how your bones and tissues grow, even your ability to make a baby. It plays a vital role in whether or not you develop diabetes, thyroid disease, growth disorders, sexual dysfunction, and a host of other hormone-related disorders.

Glands of the Endocrine System

Each gland of the endocrine system releases specific hormones into your bloodstream. These hormones travel through your blood to other cells and help control or coordinate many body processes.

Endocrine glands include:

• Adrenal glands: Two glands that sit on top of the kidneys that release the hormone cortisol.

• Hypothalamus: A part of the lower middle brain that tells the pituitary gland when to release hormones.

• Ovaries: The female reproductive organs that release eggs and produce sex hormones.

• Islet cells in the pancreas: Cells in the pancreas control the release of the hormones insulin and glucagon.

• Parathyroid: Four tiny glands in the neck that play a role in bone development.

• Pineal gland: A gland found near the center of the brain that may be linked to sleep patterns.

• Pituitary gland: A gland found at the base of brain behind the sinuses. It is often called the "master gland" because it influences many other glands, especially the thyroid. Problems with the pituitary gland can affect bone growth, a woman's menstrual cycles, and the release of breast milk.

• Testes: The male reproductive glands that produce sperm and sex hormones.

• Thymus: A gland in the upper chest that helps develop the body's immune system early in life.

• Thyroid: A butterfly-shaped gland in the front of the neck that controls metabolism.

Even the slightest hiccup with the function of one or more of these glands can throw off the delicate balance of hormones in your body and lead to an endocrine disorder, or endocrine disease.

Causes of Endocrine Disorders

There is no specific set of causes of endocrine disorders, as there are many different types of these diseases. The endocrine system, which includes the pituitary gland, thyroid gland, parathyroid gland, adrenal glands, pancreas, ovaries, and testicles, uses hormones to regulate and coordinate a range of functions in the body, including growth, reproduction, and energy level. Generally, an endocrine disorder will arise when there is a problem with the feedback system that maintains certain levels of hormones in the bloodstream. Due to the complex and interconnected nature of this system, there are a range of conditions that can result in endocrine disorders, including:

• Tumors of one or more endocrine gland

• A bodily infection that influences hormone levels

• Damage to an endocrine gland

• Genetic disorders such as familial isolated hyperparathyroidism (FIHP)

• Problems with the endocrine feedback system, causing the overproduction or underproduction of certain hormones

At Tampa General Hospital, we take a comprehensive approach to treating disorders of the endocrine system and their causes. Each patient receives an individual treatment plan tailored to his or her unique condition by our team of surgeons, endocrinologists, and other specialists. Our exceptional level of experience is evidenced by the fact that we perform more than 2,500 surgeries a year for parathyroid diseases alone.

Causes of Endocrine Disorders

Endocrine disorders are typically grouped into two categories:

• Endocrine disease that results when a gland produces too much or too little of an endocrine hormone, called a hormone imbalance.

• Endocrine disease due to the development of lesions (such as nodules or tumors) in the endocrine system, which may or may not affect hormone levels.

The endocrine's feedback system helps control the balance of hormones in the bloodstream. If your body has too much or too little of a certain hormone, the feedback system signals the proper gland or glands to correct the problem. A hormone imbalance may occur if this feedback system has trouble keeping the right level of hormones in the bloodstream, or if your body doesn't clear them out of the bloodstream properly.

Increased or decreased levels of endocrine hormone may be caused by:

• A problem with the endocrine feedback system

• Disease

• Failure of a gland to stimulate another gland to release hormones (for example, a problem with the hypothalamus can disrupt hormone production in the pituitary gland)

• A genetic disorder, such as multiple endocrine neoplasia (MEN) or congenital hypothyroidism

• Infection

• Injury to an endocrine gland

• Tumor of an endocrine gland

Most endocrine tumors and nodules (lumps) are noncancerous. They usually do not spread to other parts of the body. However, a tumor or nodule on the gland may interfere with the gland's hormone production.

Endocrine System Diseases and Disorders

Endocrine diseases and disorders result from the improper function of the endocrine system, which includes the glands that secrete hormones, the receptors that respond to the hormones, and the organs that are directly impacted by these hormones. At any one of these points, dysfunction can occur, causing wide-ranging effects on the body. Tampa General Hospital is able to diagnose and treat all types of endocrine problems, addressing their far-reaching side effects.

Named one of America's Best Hospitals for Diabetes & Endocrinology by U.S. News & World Report, TGH has the experienced physicians, caring support staff, and medical equipment necessary to treat endocrine system diseases and related issues, including but not limited to:

• Menopause – The reduction of estrogen and fluctuation of other hormones can cause a host of symptoms, including cardiovascular issues and bone problems like osteoarthritis.

• Diabetes – The body is either not producing enough insulin or isn't responding to it properly, leading to high blood sugar levels and many long-term complications.

• Metabolic disorders – Improper levels of certain hormones can alter the body's metabolism and affect its function (diabetes is an example).

• Lack of growth – Low levels or poor absorption of growth hormone can contribute to lack of proper cell reproduction and growth.

• Thyroid diseases – When the body is producing too much or too little thyroid hormone, it can affect a person's overall metabolism.

• Weight gain – Gaining weight can result from hypothyroidism, Cushing's syndrome, and other endocrine systems diseases and disorders.

• Cancers of the endocrine glands – When tumors grow within hormone-secreting glands, they can affect the production of hormones, making this type of cancer particularly complex to treat.

Types of Endocrine Disorders

There are many different types of endocrine disorders. Diabetes is the most common endocrine disorder diagnosed in the U.S.

Other endocrine disorders include:

Adrenal insufficiency. The adrenal gland releases too little of the hormone cortisol and sometimes, aldosterone. Symptoms include fatigue, stomach upset, dehydration, and skin changes. Addison's disease is a type of adrenal insufficiency.

Cushing's disease. Overproduction of a pituitary gland hormone leads to an overactive adrenal gland. A similar condition called Cushing's syndrome may occur in people, particularly children, who take high doses of corticosteroid medications.

Gigantism (acromegaly) and other growth hormone problems.

If the pituitary gland produces too much growth hormone, a child's bones and body parts may grow abnormally fast. If growth hormone levels are too low, a child can stop growing in height.

Hyperthyroidism. The thyroid gland produces too much thyroid hormone, leading to weight loss, fast heart rate, sweating, and nervousness. The most common cause for an overactive thyroid is an autoimmune disorder called Grave's disease.

Hypothyroidism. The thyroid gland does not produce enough thyroid hormone, leading to fatigue, constipation, dry skin, and depression. The underactive gland can cause slowed development in children. Some types of hypothyroidism are present at birth.

Hypopituitarism. The pituitary gland releases little or no hormones. It may be caused by a number of different diseases.

Women with this condition may stop getting their periods.

Multiple endocrine neoplasia I and II (MEN I and MEN II). These rare, genetic conditions are passed down through families. They cause tumors of the parathyroid, adrenal, and thyroid glands, leading to overproduction of hormones.

Polycystic ovary syndrome (PCOS). Overproduction of androgens interfere with the development of eggs and their release from the female ovaries. PCOS is a leading cause of infertility.

Precocious puberty. Abnormally early puberty that occurs when glands tell the body to release sex hormones too soon in life.

Testing for Endocrine Disorders

If you have an endocrine disorder, your doctor may refer you to a specialist called an endocrinologist. An endocrinologist is specially trained in problems with the endocrine system.

The symptoms of an endocrine disorder vary widely and depend on the specific gland involved. However, most people with endocrine disease complain of fatigue and weakness.

Blood and urine tests to check your hormone levels can help your doctors determine if you have an endocrine disorder. Imaging tests may be done to help locate or pinpoint a nodule or tumor.

Treatment of endocrine disorders can be complicated, as a change in one hormone level can throw off another. Your doctor or specialist may order routine blood work to check for problems or to determine if your medication or treatment plan needs to be adjusted.

Symptoms of Endocrine Disorders

There is no specific set of symptoms of endocrine disorders. This is because symptoms will vary depending on the specific kind of endocrine disease a patient has, as well as the severity of his or her condition. For example, hyperthyroidism, a disease marked by the overproduction of thyroxine in the thyroid gland, may cause sudden weight loss, tremors, anxiety, rapid heartbeat, thinning of the skin, and other symptoms. However, diseases of the parathyroid gland can result in a very different set of symptoms, such as lack of energy, depression, osteoporosis, recurrent headaches, kidney stones, and others.

Though no symptom is universal, weakness and fatigue are commonly reported and it is generally wise for patients to seek medical care upon noticing any significant change in their daily functioning. Because the endocrine system is interconnected and uses hormones to communicate with glands that control and coordinate growth, energy level, reproduction, and other functions, any changes in one gland can cause changes in another. The glands that make up the endocrine system include the:

- Pituitary gland

- Thyroid gland

- Parathyroid gland

- Pancreas

- Adrenal glands

- Ovaries (in women)

- Testicles (in men)

Patients with an endocrine disorders can visit Tampa General Hospital to receive the highest standard of care from a multispecialty team. We utilize leading-edge diagnostic, medical, and surgical technologies and techniques to accurately identify each patient's unique condition and develop an individualized treatment plan. For patients dealing with parathyroid diseases alone, we've performed more than 20,000 surgeries and, whenever possible, use minimally invasive technique to expedite recovery and reduce the likelihood of complications.

CBD for Endocrine Disorders

Endocrine disorders are health situations that happen when there is an abnormality in an endocrine gland. The endocrine system is liable for the production of hormones. Hormones are biochemical signs that are sent out through the bloodstream. Their role is to help the body in the management of several processes, which includes breathing, growth, appetite, feminization, weight control, virilization, and fluid balance. The most common "endocrine disorders" are diabetes mellitus, acromegaly, Addison's disease, Cushing's syndrome, Graves' disease, and Hashimoto's thyroiditis.

How can CBD help?

CBD oil has received tremendous attention in recent years, and the reason is its therapeutic potential. Cannabinoid or CBD have been found to demonstrate remarkable anti-anxiety, anti-inflammatory, anti-tumor, neuroprotective, and antioxidant effects, among other drugs. The more these compounds are examined, the more their mechanism of operation is explained. The cannabinoid has been observed to work in many ways within the human body, with the primary pathways relating to the endocannabinoid system, i.e., ECS.

ECS – Endocannabinoid System

The case studies show the endocannabinoid system plays a regulatory role over many other systems inside the body. The ECS is made up of two main receptors, namely CB1 and CB2 receptors, which are found on many different cell types everywhere inside the body. CBD is not the only chemicals that affect these receptors. Endocannabinoids or cannabinoids created inside the body, also stimulate these receptor sites and play a vital role in human physiology as examined areas such as mood and appetite.

One of the biological systems that the endocannabinoid system seems to influence is the "endocrine system." Research came in the year 2006 reviewing endocrine system states that CB1 receptors are manifested in the 'hypothalamus' and 'pituitary gland.' Along with their activation distinguished to change all of the endocrine hypothalamic-peripheral endocrine axes.

The presence of cannabinoid receptors inside the endocrine system suggests that CBD may have healing potential when it comes to dealing with 'endocrine disorders.'

THE ENDOCRINE SYSTEM

The endocrine system is composed of 'glands' that generate hormones inside the body. Hormones are signaling molecules transported by the circulatory system that is capable of regulating physiology and behavior.

The main elements of the endocrine system are the hypothalamus, pineal, pituitary, thyroid, thymus, adrenals, parathyroid, pancreas, and ovaries/testes. The hormones released by these glands include melatonin, insulin, testosterone, epinephrine, glucagon, and luteinizing hormone. Such hormones help to improve processes in the body, for instance, sleep, the fight or flight response, growth, energy storage, and development.

The Endocannabinoid System

The large and widespread medical, religious, and recreational use of marijuana throughout the ages was apparently not sufficient to initiate careful and extensive research on cannabinoids until the last few decades of the 20th century. Conversely, the political antimarijuana attitude in the United States and the consequent prohibition in the 1930s did not help to encourage scientific interest on this topic. In the 1960s, the growing public concern regarding the potential negative healthy effects of cannabinoids associated with the exponential increase in its recreational use forced governmental institutions to invest resources to understand the modes of action of marijuana and the pathophysiological implications of its use in more detail. Cannabinoid research received a pivotal boost from the characterization of the chemical structure of Δ9-tetrahydrocannabinol (Δ9-THC), the main psychoactive constituent of marijuana (2). This finding paved the way to the understanding of marijuana's mechanisms of action and, many years later, to the cloning of the two receptor subtypes that are able to bind exogenous cannabinoids, named cannabinoid receptor type 1 (CB1 receptor) and type 2 (CB2 receptor), respectively, and to the identification of their endogenous ligands: the endocannabinoids (5–9). Cannabinoid receptors, endocannabinoids, and the machinery for their synthesis and degradation represent the elements of a novel endogenous signaling system (the so-called endocannabinoid system), which is involved in a plethora of physiological functions (3, 4). During the last few years, an overwhelming amount of data has been acquired to understand the biological roles of this system in more detail. However, many questions are still open, and promising new discoveries await us in the near future.

In general, the endocannabinoid system is involved in many different physiological functions, many of which relate to stress-recovery systems and to the maintenance of homeostatic balance (10). Among other functions, the endocannabinoid system is involved in neuroprotection (11–13), modulation of nociception (14), regulation of motor activity (15), and the control of certain phases of memory processing (16–18). In addition, the endocannabinoid system is involved in modulating the immune and inflammatory responses (19–21). It also influences the cardiovascular and respiratory systems by controlling heart rate, blood pressure, and bronchial functions (22). Finally, yet importantly, endocannabinoids are known to exert important antiproliferative actions in tumor cells (23). A full discussion of the plethora of functions of the endocannabinoid system in maintaining homeostasis is beyond the scope and space of the present review. However, the reviews cited in this article will further help to obtain a broad insight into the physiological roles of the endocannabinoid system.

Cannabidiol (CBD)

This brings us to the cannabinoid du jour, cannabidiol or CBD. Long playing the second fiddle to the more active tetrahydrocannabinol (THC). CBD does not interact strongly with either the CB1 or CB2 receptors. Instead, it is able to increase endocannabinoid tone by inhibiting fatty acid amide hydrolase (FAAH), and enzyme that breaks down cannabinoids in the body. FAAH inhibitors may be may be helpful for people with anxiety-related disorders because they appear to improve the regulation of the HPA axis. It's unknown precisely how this happens, how this happens but it appears they help to modulate the sensitivity of the cannabinoid receptors in the body.in the body.

In addition to its stimulatory effects on HPA, the ECS also plays a critical inhibitory role in regulating HPA functions. Researchers found that endocannabinoid signaling negatively modulates the stress-induced activation of the HPA axis, confirming the notion that an increase in endocannabinoid signaling activity may constitute a novel approach to improving the lives of people with anxiety-related disorders.

Currently, the best way to boost endocannabinoid signaling, improve the regulation of the HPA, and promote a healthy endocrine system is the use of a dietary cannabinoid supplement made from hemp. These products contain naturally occurring cannabinoids, including CBD, which have been shown to naturally increase ECS tone which helps to improve the regulation of homeostasis across the HPA axis. This will improve both the physiological and psychological responses to stress making us more likely to resist the cascade that leads to HPA dysfunction and endocrine-related health problems. Enjoy a cannabinoid supplement every day!

Conclusion

CBD may be able to aid with the symptoms of endocrine disorders. CBD is a non-psychoactive component of the cannabis plant that manifests various medicinal treatments. Side effects of some endocrine disorders are anxiety and insomnia. CBD is well-known to decrease feelings of anxiety, as documented in human case studies. The CBD may also help with improving sleep patterns by decreasing stress and enhancing REM sleep.

Cannabinoids are the derivatives of the cannabis plant, the most potent bioactive component of which is tetrahydrocannabinol (THC). The most commonly used drugs containing cannabinoids are marijuana, hashish, and hashish oil. These compounds exert their effects via interaction with the cannabinoid receptors CB1 and CB2. Type 1 receptors (CB1) are localised mostly in the central nervous system and in the adipose tissue and many visceral organs, including most endocrine organs. Type 2 cannabinoid receptors (CB2) are positioned in the peripheral nervous system (peripheral nerve endings) and on the surface of the immune system cells. Recently, more and more attention has been paid to the role that endogenous ligands play for these receptors, as well as to the role of the receptors themselves. So far, endogenous cannabinoids have been confirmed to participate in the regulation of food intake and energy homeostasis of the body, and have a significant impact on the endocrine system, including the activity of the pituitary gland, adrenal cortex, thyroid gland, pancreas, and gonads. Interrelations between the endocannabinoid system and the activity of the endocrine system may be a therapeutic target for a number of drugs that have been proved effective in the treatment of infertility, obesity, diabetes, and even prevention of diseases associated with the cardiovascular system.

Where should I buy CBD oil from?

CBD industry is unregulated. This has given rise to many companies who provide fake products. We want you to be healthy and safe while using CBD oils. We use CO2 extraction to guarantee purity. Our products are not just natural but also 100% safe.

A. Cannabinoid receptors

Two cannabinoid receptors have been identified and molecularly characterized so far, namely the seven transmembrane G protein-coupled cannabinoid receptor type 1 (CB1 receptor) (6) and type 2 (CB2 receptor) (7). CB1 receptor was originally described as the "brain type" cannabinoid receptor, because its levels of expression were high in the brain (24). However, recent studies attribute new sites of action of endocannabinoids to many peripheral organs through CB1 receptor activation. The generalization for CB1 receptor being the eminent "brain type" receptor is therefore no longer appropriate. Conversely, CB2 receptors are present almost exclusively in immune and blood cells, where they may participate in regulating immune responses (25). However, CB2 receptors also exert functions in nonimmune cells such as keratinocytes (26). Pharmacological evidence exists for the presence of other cannabinoid receptors, which, however, have not yet been cloned (27). The endocannabinoid anandamide is also able to bind to and activate vanilloid receptors, transient receptor potential vanilloid type 1 (28), and to inhibit TASK-1 K+ channels (29). Moreover, pharmacological studies indicate that still unidentified additional cannabinoid receptors might exist in the hippocampus, modulating the release of glutamate (30), and on endothelial cells (31). Two patents have been recently published claiming that a number of cannabinoid ligands also bind to GPR55, an orphan G protein-coupled receptor, suggesting that this receptor might represent a novel target of cannabinoid action (32). CB1 receptor, however, is the best characterized target of exogenous and endogenous cannabinoids in the modulation of neuroendocrine and metabolic responses, and this review will focus mainly on this receptor.

1. CB1 receptor expression in the brain

Cannabinoid receptor distribution was studied by means of autoradiography of ligand-receptor binding on slide-mounted rat brain sections (24, 33), by in situ hybridization (ISH) (34–36), by autoradiography in human brain (37), by immunohistochemistry (IHC) (38–41), and by agonist-stimulated [35S]GTPγS binding to slide-mounted sections (42, 43). Expression studies showed very early that CB1 receptor is one of the most abundant G protein-coupled receptors in the mammalian brain (24). CB1 receptors are widely expressed in the brain, including the olfactory bulb, cortical regions (neocortex, pyriform cortex, hippocampus, and amygdala), several parts of basal ganglia, thalamic and hypothalamic nuclei, cerebellar cortex, and brainstem nuclei. The levels of expression vary considerably among the various brain regions and neuronal subpopulations. For instance, agonist-mediated receptor binding revealed high densities of CB1 receptor protein in the cornu ammonis pyramidal cell layers of the hippocampus (24), which was later shown by IHC to be due to a dense plexus of immunoreactive fibers deriving from γ-aminobutyric acid (GABA)-ergic interneurons and surrounding the cell bodies of pyramidal cells, which appear per se to be devoid of CB1 receptor protein (38, 41, 44). However, pyramidal cells of the hippocampus and other cortical regions do express low but significant levels of CB1 receptor mRNA (34, 36), indicating the possibility that CB1 receptor protein in these cells is localized on distal projections and/or is expressed at low levels, which are below the limit of detectability with currently available immunohistochemical methods. A similar situation is present also in other cortical regions, such as the amygdala, neocortex, entorhinal cortex, and piriform cortex.

In subcortical regions, CB1 receptor is present at relatively high levels in the septal region (lateral and medial septum, and vertical and horizontal nuclei of the diagonal band). Lower levels of expression are present in hypothalamic regions, such as the medial and lateral preoptic nucleus, magnocellular preoptic nucleus, and paraventricular nucleus (PVN) (36). In the caudal hypothalamus, CB1 receptor is expressed in the premammillary nucleus. In the lateral hypothalamus, CB1 receptor is present in scattered cells (34, 36). In the PVN, CB1 receptor mRNA coexpresses with CRH mRNA (45). In the thalamus, CB1 receptor is present in the lateral habenula, reticular thalamic nucleus, and zona incerta. Midbrain dopaminergic neurons are generally considered to lack CB1 receptor expression. However, recent observations indicate that very low levels of CB1 receptor might be present in tyrosine hydroxylase-expressing neurons in the ventral tegmental area (VTA) (46) and in dopaminergic terminals in the striatum (47). In the hindbrain, apart from the molecular and granular layers of cerebellum expressing high levels of the receptor, CB1 receptor is present at low levels in some nuclei of the brain stem, such as the periaqueductal gray (34, 38). Functional mapping by agonist-stimulated [35S]GTPγS binding using different CB1 receptor agonists revealed that cannabinoid activation of G proteins occurs with the same regional distribution as the receptors (43, 48). However, in some regions, the ratio between the estimated amount of CB1 receptor and G protein activation is not always constant, thus indicating regional differences in receptor-coupling efficiencies (43). This is important to consider, because sometimes the endocannabinoid system seems to influence functions involving regions where the density of CB1 receptor is relatively low (e.g., modulation of food intake in the hypothalamic area). Therefore, the activity of cannabinoids on CB1 receptor cannot be predicted based solely on the relative receptor density, but other factors, such as receptor coupling efficiency, should be taken into account. For instance, by using conditional mutagenesis in mice, the relatively low levels of CB1 receptor expression in cortical pyramidal neurons were recently shown to play a central role in the endocannabinoid-mediated protection against excitotoxic seizures (12). In conclusion, CB1 receptor is widely expressed in the brain and is present at different levels in different neuronal subpopulation and brain regions, and there is apparently no strict correlation between levels of expression and receptor functionality.

2. CB1 receptor expression in the pituitary

Early studies showed a scattered presence of CB1 receptor in both lobes of the rodent pituitary (33). Recent studies examined the distribution of CB1 receptor mRNA in the anterior pituitary lobe in more detail. In 1999, the abundant CB1 receptor presence in the rat adenohypophysis was associated with the ability of this gland to synthesize endocannabinoids (49). CB1 receptor was also shown to be present in prolactin (PRL)- and LH-secreting cells of the rat pituitary (50). CB1 receptor expression was also detected by means of double-immunofluorescence in the pituitary gland of Xenopus laevis, where the receptor was found in lactotrophs, gonadotrophs, and thyrotrophs (51). The expression of CB1 receptor in the human pituitary appears to be substantially different from the localization of the same receptor described in rodents and frogs (52). By using ISH and double IHC, CB1 receptor was localized in the majority of corticotrophs and somatotrophs of the normal human anterior lobe; only a small percentage of the PRL-secreting cells are positive for CB1 receptor, whereas no immunoreactivity was found in LH-, FSH-, or TSH-positive cells. The neural lobe is devoid of CB1 receptor immunoreactivity (52). Interestingly, folliculo-stellate cells are also positive for CB1 receptor, although functional data have not yet been associated with this expression (52). CB1 receptor was also found in human pituitary adenomas, such as ACTH-producing adenomas (which give rise to Cushing's syndrome), GH-producing tumors (leading to acromegaly), and in prolactinomas, whereas no CB1 receptor staining was found in so-called nonfunctioning pituitary adenomas, tumors expressing LH and/or

FSH, and/or α-subunit being devoid of any hormonal staining (52). These data were confirmed by a study in which cDNA microarray analysis was used to compare gene expression pattern in pituitary adenomas vs. normal pituitary (53). Among other genes differentially expressed, ACTH- and GH-producing tumors express higher levels of CB1 receptor compared with the normal pituitary . Notably, the human normal anterior pituitary gland and pituitary tumors were shown to be capable of synthesizing endocannabinoids .

In rodents, CB1 receptor expression in the pituitary is under the influence of circulating sex hormones, as demonstrated by the ability of androgens and estrogens to up- and down-regulate CB1 receptor, respectively. In agreement with these findings, decreased CB1 receptor expression has been found in estrogen-induced pituitary hyperplasia in rats. Accordingly, in rats, the male pituitary displays higher levels of CB1 receptor mRNA than the female one (49). In contrast, the human pituitary does not show this gender difference .

Exogenous cannabinoids can modulate the expression of CB1 receptor in the pituitary. After a transient down-regulation of the receptor (first 1–3 d), chronic administration of CB1 receptor agonists is able to produce a consistent increase of CB1 receptor expression in the anterior pituitary lobe (after 14 d) (54). This finding seems to be in contrast with the level in the ventromedial hypothalamic nucleus, where CB1 receptor mRNA was down-regulated by chronic CB1 receptor agonist treatment .

3. CB1 receptor expression in the peripheral organs

a. CB1 receptor in the thyroid gland

CB1 receptor expression during the late embryological stages of the rat thyroid was found to be very high , whereas lower but still detectable levels of CB1 receptor mRNA and protein were present in the adult rat gland distributed in both follicular and parafollicular cells as demonstrated by IHC .

b. CB1 receptor in the adrenal gland

A faint signal for CB1 receptor was detected in the human adrenal glands by quantitative RT-PCR method . However, ISH or IHC studies are needed to clearly localize CB1 receptor in the different areas that make up the gland.

c. CB1 receptor in the peripheral organs involved in metabolic control

In 2003, two independent groups found the presence of CB1 receptor in adipocytes of mice and humans . In both species, this expression is more evident in mature adipocytes than in preadipocytes, indicating that the full cellular machinery of the fat cell is needed to exert cannabinoid action. Little is known about CB1 receptor expression in the muscle. Recently, the

CB1 receptor antagonist SR141716 was shown to directly affect glucose uptake in the isolated soleus muscle of genetically obese mice .Consistently, CB1 receptor is present in the murine soleus muscle.Additional investigations are needed to fully understand the importance of this expression site.

CBD AND THE ENDOCRINE SYSTEM

CBD may have the potential to manage the endocrine system and support with cases of specific endocrine disorders. These compounds may be useful in treating endocrine disorders caused by the presence of tumors on certain endocrine glands. A 2008 case study for Cancer states that endocannabinoids can inhibit cell growth, metastasis of thyroid, invasion, breast, and prostate tumors. Because cannabinoids such as THC also activate the same receptors due to the similarity in molecular composition, they may be able to deliver similar results.

Research has also shown the existence of cannabinoid receptors on nerves involved in the regulation of the hypothalamic-pituitary-thyroid axis. This region controls the creation of hormones through the thyroid gland, advising that endocannabinoids and CBD may have influence over hormone production. Research in this area is introductory, but it indicates that CBD may be able to regulate the 'endocrine system.'

CBD TO RELIEVE ENDOCRINE DISORDERS

The use of CBD as a relief supplement for endocrine disorders is based on the severity of a patient's symptoms. In some cases, patients exhibit mild symptoms that do not need immediate therapeutic aid. Usually, symptoms occur when the body produces excess hormones, or in some cases a deficit amount. The first strategy is ideally to correct the hormonal imbalance if the symptoms are bothersome. This is usually done through the administration of a synthetic hormone.

CBD AS A THERAPEUTIC AID FOR ENDOCRINE DISORDERS

The body's natural endocannabinoid system plays a role in the regulation of the activities of the body including homeostasis. Researchers have found that endocannabinoid molecules have anti-carcinogenic effects on thyroid tumors through animal studies. Endocannabinoid receptors are found in regions of the brain that send signals to the thyroid gland which produces many hormones.

A study published in the Journal of Endocrinology in 2009 reported that there are many CB1 receptors in the brain nerves, and that they are involved in the hypothalamic-pituitary-thyroid axis as well as its regulation. This is the area that controls hormone production by the thyroid gland, and this distribution shows great inhibitory and excitatory input potential.

WHY USE CBD FOR ENDOCRINE DISORDERS?

The urinary tract is in charge of the legislation of human hormones that control hunger, metabolism, and moods among other body techniques. CBD may be used to appropriate different endocrine disorders by regulating the endocannabinoid system. A significant after effect of CBD on the urinary tract is lessening cortisol level in bloodstream plasma. When there is a low degree of cortisol, one has reduced stress which helps prevent diseases that are triggered by stress. On top of that, CBD lessens the amount of fear, anxiety, and anxiousness. Nevertheless, people who have endocrine disorders should speak to their doctors before they use CBD to alleviate them.

HOW IT WORKS

Recent preclinical research has indicated the importance of ensuring the health of the endocannabinoid system in the therapeutic aid of endocrine disorders. That's because when the endocannabinoid system has a healthy tone, a person has better stress resilience as well as reduced residual post-traumatic anxiety, panic behaviors, and fears.

Studies show that CBD reduces anxiety. That's because it activates receptors outside CB2. These include

TRPV1 and 5HT1A. These are involved in mitigating fear or panic response to stress and can act as an anxiolytic. Currently, there is adequate scientific evidence that proves the essence of maintaining a healthy endocannabinoid system when it comes to relieving endocrine disorders. CBD helps in maintaining this system. Emerging clinical data and preclinical data supports the use of CBD products in modulating anxiety, fear, and in promoting a healthy response to stress, which leads to the production of hormones.

USING CBD TO RELIEVE ENDOCRINE DISORDERS

The endocrine system is responsible for the regulation of hormones that control appetite, metabolism, and mood among other bodily processes. CBD can be used to correct different endocrine disorders by regulating the endocannabinoid system. The major effect of CBD on the endocrine system is decreasing cortisol level in blood plasma. When there is a low level of cortisol, a person has reduced stress and this prevents severe conditions that are caused by stress. Additionally, CBD lessens the level of fear, panic, and anxiety in patients. Nevertheless, people with endocrine disorders should talk to their doctors before they use CBD to relieve them.

The Role of the Endocannabinoid System in Restoring Balance to the Endocrine System

Over the last few years, cannabis and the endocannabinoid system have emerged as a topic of interest among both patients and within the scientific community. The involvement of endocannabinoids in several diseases and conditions where the suspected cause is an underlying physiological dysfunction has attracted intense scrutiny. The endogenous cannabinoid system (ECS), named after the cannabis plant that led to its discovery, is one of the most important physiological system involved in establishing and maintaining human health. Endocannabinoids and their receptors, CB1 and CB2, are found throughout the body: in the brain, organs, connective tissues, glands, and immune cells. In each tissue, the ECS performs different tasks with the goal of maintaining homeostasis, the maintenance of a stable internal environment despite fluctuations in the external environment.

The Endocrine System

The endocrine system is the collection of glands in the body that secrete hormones into the bloodstream to be carried towards distant target organs. The central neuroendocrine systems is the interface between the brain and the rest of the endocrine systems. The part of the brain that balances the release of hormones in the body is called the hypothalamus and sits right on top of the pituitary gland where it regulates stress, metabolism, growth, reproduction, and lactation. All of these processes are regulated by the hypothalamus releasing or inhibiting the release of hormones by the pituitary gland. The release of pituitary hormones affects downstream physiological functions. Other hypothalamic neuroendocrine cells control water/salt balance, and lactation and childbirth, through the release of vasopressin and oxytocin. Together, these hypothalamic neuroendocrine functions enable the central nervous system to respond rapidly to internal or external environmental change, and to maintain a response through endocrine hormonal transducers. The endocannabinoid system modulates the regulation of the neuroendocrine system, which regulates organ function and stress response and helps maintain a healthy balance across the neuroendocrine system and related physiological body system.

The endocrine system is the collection of glands in the body that secrete hormones into the bloodstream to be carried towards distant target organs. The central neuroendocrine system is the interface between the brain and the rest of the endocrine systems. The hypothalamus is the part of the brain that balances the release or inhibition of release of hormones in the body. The hypothalamus sits right on top of the pituitary gland which releases hormones that regulate stress, metabolism, growth, reproduction, and lactation. The function of the central neuroendocrine system, including the hypothalamus and pituitary gland, is to enable the central nervous system to respond rapidly to internal or external environmental change and to maintain a response through endocrine hormonal transducers. The ECS modulates the regulation of the neuroendocrine system, which regulates organ function and stress response and helps maintain a healthy balance across the neuroendocrine system and related physiological body system.

Targeting the Endocannabinoid System for Endocrine Regulation

Cannabinoids in cannabis have long been known to be able to affect the secretion of pituitary hormones. By way of the ECS we regulate our hormonal balance, both up and down, through a direct effect on the organs themselves. The stimulation of the hypothalamic-pituitary-adrenal (HPA) axis is a crucial neuroendocrine response to stress and is dependent on CB1 receptor-mediated signaling. Activating the CB1 receptors in the hypothalamus results in a signaling cascade that ultimately inhibits overall neuroendocrine function. Stress is well known to affect endocrine function and a poorly regulated endocrine system can lead to major health problems. The endocrine response, as part of the HPA axis, is central to its regulation.

Up until a few years ago, the stimulatory effects of cannabinoids on the HPA axis was considered as an exception. The commonly accepted view of the ECS was that it played a general inhibitory role on neuroendocrine functions. We now understand that cannabinoids can have both stimulatory and inhibitory effects on the HPA axis which is how it's able to modulate its regulation. These biphasic effects of cannabinoids, both stimulatory and inhibitory, are increasingly revealing themselves as we look closer at the interactions between the ECS and the endocrine system.

Cannabidiol (CBD)

This brings us to the cannabinoid du jour, cannabidiol or CBD. Long playing the second fiddle to the more active tetrahydrocannabinol (THC). CBD does not interact strongly with either the CB1 or CB2 receptors. Instead, it is able to increase endocannabinoid tone by inhibiting fatty acid amide hydrolase (FAAH), and enzyme that breaks down cannabinoids in the body. FAAH inhibitors may be may be helpful for people with anxiety-related disorders because they appear to improve the regulation of the HPA axis. It's unknown precisely how this happens, how this happens but it appears they help to modulate the sensitivity of the cannabinoid receptors in the body.in the body.

In addition to its stimulatory effects on HPA, the ECS also plays a critical inhibitory role in regulating HPA functions. Researchers found that endocannabinoid signaling negatively modulates the stress-induced activation of the HPA axis, confirming the notion that an increase in endocannabinoid signaling activity may constitute a novel approach to improving the lives of people with anxiety-related disorders.

Currently, the best way to boost endocannabinoid signaling, improve the regulation of the HPA, and promote a healthy endocrine system is the use of a dietary cannabinoid supplement made from hemp. These products contain naturally occurring cannabinoids, including CBD, which have been shown to naturally increase ECS tone which helps to improve the regulation of homeostasis across the HPA axis. This will improve both the physiological and psychological responses to stress making us more likely to resist the cascade that leads to HPA dysfunction and endocrine-related health problems. Enjoy a cannabinoid supplement every day!

Conclusion

CBD may be able to aid with the symptoms of endocrine disorders. CBD is a non-psychoactive component of the cannabis plant that manifests various medicinal treatments. Side effects of some endocrine disorders are anxiety and insomnia. CBD is well-known to decrease feelings of anxiety, as documented in human case studies. The CBD may also help with improving sleep patterns by decreasing stress and enhancing REM sleep.

Cannabinoids are the derivatives of the cannabis plant, the most potent bioactive component of which is tetrahydrocannabinol (THC). The most commonly used drugs containing cannabinoids are marijuana, hashish, and hashish oil. These compounds exert their effects via interaction with the cannabinoid receptors CB1 and CB2. Type 1 receptors (CB1) are localised mostly in the central nervous system and in the adipose tissue and many visceral organs, including most endocrine organs. Type 2 cannabinoid receptors (CB2) are positioned in the peripheral nervous system (peripheral nerve endings) and on the surface of the immune system cells. Recently, more and more attention has been paid to the role that endogenous ligands play for these receptors, as well as to the role of the receptors themselves. So far, endogenous cannabinoids have been confirmed to participate in the regulation of food intake and energy homeostasis of the body, and have a significant impact on the endocrine system, including the activity of the pituitary gland, adrenal cortex, thyroid gland, pancreas, and gonads. Interrelations between the endocannabinoid system and the activity of the endocrine system may be a therapeutic target for a number of drugs that have been proved effective in the treatment of infertility, obesity, diabetes, and even prevention of diseases associated with the cardiovascular system.

Where should I buy CBD oil from?

CBD industry is unregulated. This has given rise to many companies who provide fake products. We want you to be healthy and safe while using CBD oils. We use CO_2 extraction to guarantee purity. Our products are not just natural but also 100% safe.